Y O GUIDE THROUGH HER BREAST CANCER JOURNEY

KATHERINE FORMOSA BOWN

First published in 2012 by Urban Traffic Publishing
www.urbantraffic.co.uk

Typeset and cover designed by Chandler Book Design
www.chandlerbookdesign.co.uk

Printed in the United Kingdom

First Printing, 2012

ISBN 978-0-9573838-0-7

This book is dedicated to my Husband Rhodri,
my Parents and my Sister Ann-Marie

I wish I knew even half of what I know now, if only to have
made your journey through my cancer a little easier!

About this Book

Since being diagnosed in 2009, I've regularly been asked by newly diagnosed women for tips and information on my experience. I've also been there to support friends and family members of recently diagnosed women, giving them an insight into my experience and how they could offer their support. I'm sure you can imagine; the news is shocking enough to take in, never mind where to start and what to do next.

Although men can be diagnosed with breast cancer, this book is aimed at those who know a female going through this journey, as I am unsure as to how the treatment affects men. I also can't stress enough that diagnosis and treatment affects people in different ways but I've put together this book giving snippets of information on how your *friend, wife, sister, mother or your loved-one* will probably react, how *you* can help and how events affected me when I was going through the cancer treatment.

I'm no medical expert and by no means do I claim to be, any recommendations I have in this book needs to be checked out by the patient's doctor, and the advice I give is from my own experience of events. This book is purely to guide you through how *you* can help based on my cancer journey, in 2009.

I really hope this book makes *your* experience of *her* breast cancer journey easier to understand and stops you feeling helpless, like so many people do.

Katherine Formosa Bown

CONTENTS

1

Preparation

I've written this book to help you understand *her* breast cancer experience and to not be a support to *your* feelings.

That probably sounds a little harsh but as I was the cancer patient myself, I only know how she's feeling, and right now I know she can't let herself begin to imagine how you feel. And although she'd be there for you in a flash if ever you were upset; she now can't be as her positivity and effort has to go *all* to herself.

Let's Get This Important Bit Out Of The Way

It'd be obvious to say that she cares about you a lot and it breaks her heart to ever see you upset, so imagine how she'd feel seeing you so upset with her being the reason? That's why positivity is key at this stage, so you need to mask those fears from her and use another friend or loved-one to offload your emotions and fears onto, as she can't see you crumble.

There may be days when she feels low, self-pity, bitter, scared, basically just awful and unfortunately for you, you have to let her ride it out. She'll go through a whole rollercoaster of emotions through the cancer journey, mainly fear and like how I reacted; she probably won't let anyone see those emotions. So there'll be days when she just wants to be left alone and these are the key times that she needs to get those emotions out, so if she's hiding in a cupboard or staring out into space whilst sat in the garden; let her, don't disturb her and most of all, just be ready for when she needs you.

My Experience

Being diagnosed made me really think about the fact that it was happening to just me, 'my' body and me. I was the only one who could truly help myself through it and I had to try and keep positive and focused at all times as I knew that if I was allowed to crumble; I'd never get the energy back to get through it.

So I masked my emotions from my friends and family, so they could mask theirs to me.

It possibly sounds quite strange to you if you've never experienced being told that you have a life-threatening illness, but the thought of dying was realisation that it would be just me dying, alone. So I had to be selfish and from the moment I was diagnosed, I went into 'Superwoman' mode!

How You Can Help

- At this point and throughout her whole breast cancer experience, you have to hold it together and put on your most 'Oscar worthy' acting role when she's around and most of all... hold back those tears!

- It's a good idea for you to suggest that she writes a blog or journal to offload her emotions, it doesn't need to be anything that someone else can read but its good to have a way to offload, as sometimes she might not want to talk to anyone about how she's really feeling.

2

Diagnosis

Hearing the confirmation that you have cancer has to be one of the most frightening things to ever hear.

She could react in any of a number of ways; staying indoors and crying it out, numb in shock and not wanting to talk about it or like how I reacted; acting like I was Superwoman and not phased by the situation. No matter what her reaction is, let her go with her emotions.

My Experience

My Superwoman reaction resulted in me carrying on at work, brushing off any sympathetic comments from well wishers saying that I was going to be alright and not to worry, and then releasing my tears and fears in the shower where no one could hear or see me.

*Looking back, I must have looked like a crazy fool;
pretending it was nothing serious but it
was the only way I could cope with the news
and I'm now grateful that I was allowed to
indulge in my madness.*

*I also, like most newly diagnosed cancer patients,
turned to fundraising. I felt that people who
donated to charities for cancer research were
about to save my life. Thankfully those people who
kindly donated, allowed the research companies
to have enough funding to investigate the best
treatments and ongoing medication in order to
saves lives, including mine, so I felt I wanted to
give something back. Don't be too surprised if she
starts fundraising, besides it'll be a great idea for
her to focus and take her mind off the reality that is
about to commence.*

I think one of the worst experiences of being diagnosed is
having to tell people who you care about that you have cancer;
especially those who didn't even know about the lump, the tests
or the hell that you've just been through waiting for the results.
And even worse than that is the bleeping sound of text after text
from concerned friends and family members, which are obviously
from caring people, but when I was diagnosed I couldn't look at
my phone for days; seeing the messages coming in made the
situation so real, and all I wanted to do was hide underneath the
bed and hoped that it would all go away!

How You Can Help

If you're one of the first to hear about the diagnosis, offer to pass on the news and tell people. If you're a family member, tell their Aunts and Uncles and ask them to pass the information down to their siblings. If you're a friend, then call their closest friends and email their acquaintances.

Some things to remember to tell them:

- To not contact her for a few days.

- To contact you direct if they have any questions.

- That you'll give them an update once you've heard any more news.

- To not post anything onto social media sites as not everyone has been informed.

Also, it's usually harder for other people to mention the cancer when they see her, which could make her feel awkward by them not mentioning it at all. So tell them to try to treat her as normal as they can, and to ask questions, it's happening, so there's no point avoiding the conversation!

My Experience

I created a private Facebook group called 'Keeping up with Kath' and invited friends to join. I used this site to post the date for my operation, chemotherapy appointments etc. so that I didn't

*need to reply to every text message/email that I
had, asking the same questions from
concerned friends.*

*With regards to people not mentioning the 'C'
word; it was just after I was diagnosed that I
attended a sporting event where we were in a
hospitality box with my husband's work colleagues.
No one mentioned the cancer, some avoided
speaking to me all together and I felt really self-
conscious. Then a few hours later once the
complimentary alcohol had been drunk, people
began to approach me and ask how I was feeling,
with one man saying 'I'm so relieved to speak
to you about it, I've felt awkward all day so the
elephant has finally left the room!'.*

*It may sound normal to you if you've never been
diagnosed or had an illness, but at the time it did
make me feel alienated from everyone in the room.*

3

Understanding Breast Cancer

I don't want to go into too much detail on medical information on tumours, mainly because I don't want to give you the wrong information.

However what I am confident is saying is that she will be 'Staged' and 'Graded' to be able to give her the best possible treatment, and here's a brief explanation:

> Please note: The text below is based on widely available information* in the UK and may differ in other countries.
> *As of July 2012

Stages

Stages range from 1 – 4 depending on the size of the tumour and whether its spread, and if so, to where.

If there is no tumour in the breast but cancer has been found in the lymph nodes in the armpit and:

- Are **not** stuck together and **no** signs of spreading to the other parts of the body – this is called Stage 2A.
- **Are** stuck together and **no** signs of spreading to the other parts of the body – this is called Stage 3A.

If the tumour size is 2cm in size or smaller and:

- **Hasn't** spread to the armpit's lymph nodes – this is called Stage 1.
- **Has** spread to the armpit's lymph nodes but are **not** stuck together and **no** signs of spreading to the other parts of the body – this is called Stage 2A.

If the tumour size is between 2cm and 5cm in size and:

- **Hasn't** spread to the armpit's lymph nodes – this is called Stage 2A.
- **Has** spread to the armpit's lymph nodes but are **not** stuck together and **no** signs of spreading to the other parts of the body – this is called Stage 2B.
- **Has** spread to the armpit's lymph nodes which **are** stuck together – this is called Stage 3A.

If the tumour size is bigger than 5cm in size and:

- **Hasn't** spread to the armpit's lymph nodes – this is called Stage 2B.
- **Has** spread to the armpit's lymph nodes and **no** signs of spreading to the other parts of the body – this is called Stage 3A.

Also:

■ If the cancer **has** spread to the breast tissue **and** possibly attached to the muscle or surrounding skin – this is called Stage 3B.

■ If the cancer **has** spread to the arm pit's lymph nodes **and** below the breastbone, above or underneath the collarbone – this is called Stage 3C.

■ If the cancer **has** spread to other body parts i.e. bones, liver, lungs etc. this is commonly known as secondary breast cancer and is called Stage 4.

Grades

The grades are based on the growth of cancer cells and how they are different to breast cells.

Grade 1 – These are cancer cells that look similar to normal cells so tend to grow slowly.

Grade 2 – These cancer cells look abnormal against normal cells and are growing a little faster than normal cells.

Grade 3 – These cancer cells look a lot different from normal cells and they tend to grow a little quicker than normal cells.

I'm sure the first thing you want to do is take to the Internet and start researching breast cancer. However I'd recommend you only stick to well-known national charities, foundations and trusts (See the Appendix for a list of websites you may find useful).

Please note that there as some scary websites out there, not to mention the images of horrific scenes that I saw when I 'Googled' for more information on breast cancer when I was diagnosed. And not once did I see such horrors during my experience, so don't go too deep into online research!

4

Surgery

Depending on the size, grade and location of the tumour, the surgeon will decide on whether a lumpectomy (Tumour removed along with surrounding tissue) or mastectomy (Removal of the breast) is required.

I had a lumpectomy therefore I can only explain about my experience. And as I previously mentioned, I'm not a medical expert therefore this is my understanding of the surgery I received:

The surgeon will remove the tumour under general anesthetic and will also take a 'healthy looking' margin around the tumour. This 'healthy looking' margin is sent for investigation to see if a miniscule cancer cell has started to spread and grow away from the tumour. If this 'healthy' margin is clear of cancer, no further surgery is required. However if there is a trace of a cancerous cell, the surgeon will need to go back and take another 'healthy looking' margin around that cell to see how far it has spread, and to keep taking it away until it is fully removed.

My Experience

Someone described this to me as the tumour being like a spider's body and the stray cancer cells are like the spider's legs. So they snip away around the 'spider's body' to see if there are any 'legs' growing off it.

Lymph Nodes

Lymph Nodes (More commonly referred to as 'glands') filter out lymphatic fluid and retain healthy cells in the body and are also responsible for detecting and rejecting foreign visitors (i.e. bacteria, viruses etc.) that may be trying to make their way through the body. They work hand in hand with the immune system and often swell or become inflamed when the body is fighting off infection. Have you ever had swollen glands in your neck when you've had cold or a throat infection? If so, then you'll know that next time your glands feel swollen, this is your lymph nodes at work!

During the operation, the surgeon will usually inject a blue dye near the tumour. The dye flows through the lymph ducts to the lymph nodes (Near the armpit) and the first few lymph nodes to turn blue are removed. This mimics the natural flow of where the cancer would spread; so the first few nodes are removed and investigated to see if the cancer has spread to the lymphatic system (Increasing the risk of spreading through the body). If the nodes are clear, no further investigation is required.

This procedure will leave a scar in the armpit and it could take about a week or so to get the results on whether the lymph nodes are clear.

My Experience

My surgery was approx. 2 hours and I stayed in hospital for 24 hours after surgery, before being discharged. I received the results of the lymph nodes examination approx. 7 days after the surgery.

Lymphoedema

After the first few lymph nodes are removed from the armpit it makes it harder for the fluid in the arms to flow to the chest, where it can get back into the bloodstream. If the remaining nodes cannot remove enough of the fluid in the area, the excess fluid builds up.

The most common symptom is swelling of the arm (Including the hand and fingers) on the side where she has been operated.

If this does happen, advise her to seek medical advice.

How You Can Help

- ■ If you're at the hospital, be prepared for the tears to flow after surgery (Mainly relief that the tumour had been taken out of her body).

- ■ Buy a skin brush and advise her to brush from her wrist up along the arm towards the shoulder, to stimulate lymph flow in the skin and reduce the risk of lymphoedema.

- ■ Make sure she's aware that due to this surgery, she should avoid:

  - Lifting anything heavy with the arm on the side she was operated on.

  - Having injections in, or taking blood from the arm on the side where she was operated on.

  - To be extra cautious for skin irritations, cuts and sun burning on this side – the lymphatic system helps to clear infections, so where the average person doesn't blink at a scratch on the arm as the lymphatic system does all of the work to heal it, she'll need to treat it quickly so keep a tube of antiseptic cream to hand.

5

Chemotherapy

A little information *(My version!)* regarding chemotherapy; it kills fast growing cells in your body however it doesn't know the difference between cancer cells and healthy cells so *every* fast growing cell is affected, this includes your white blood cells (Which you need for fighting infection) therefore the immune system will need to be closely monitored!

My Experience

The chemotherapy I had was FEC (FEC-ing chemo, I couldn't believe it!), which stands for Fluorouracil (5FU), Epirubicin and Cyclophosphamide (I did have to 'Google' that part!).

It was administered intravenously into my hand (I actually feel sick right now typing this part – 3 years later!) and there was so much of it that the nurse arrived with 6 comedy-sized syringes (2 for F, 2 for E and 2 for C). Each one giving a different sensation as it was administered: one felt cold in my veins, one felt warm and the other gave me a twitchy nose!).

The chemo was given on week 1 where I fell into my 'chemo coma', week 2 was where my immune system was down, so this was the week that I could possibly catch an infection, and then week 3 where my white blood cells would grow, making my body strong enough to be ready for the next treatment of chemotherapy. This cycle went on for 18 weeks (6 rounds of chemo).

My Chemotherapy Cycle

Chemo 1

I suffered with nausea, felt exhausted and I craved salted flavoured foods including crisps, chips and crackers. My mouth went from a sickly watery taste to feeling like there was metal in my mouth and I ate ice-lollies to rehydrate (I found that the supermarket's own brand of cheap ice-lollies were the best as they didn't have a strong taste).

Chemo 2

My second was a weird one; no sickness (Phew!) I just felt like I'd swum across the Atlantic Ocean, and drank it! I was exhausted, too exhausted to get up; my arms ached, I felt dizzy going upstairs and my mouth tasted of sea water so I couldn't eat anything; ice-lollies came up trumps again!

Before Chemo 3 I took a holiday in the sunshine to Spain with 3 friends; total bliss and I felt human again, if only for a week!

Chemo 3

Extreme fatigue, ulcers, cold sores and dry skin.

Chemo Number 4

A knock out, I was so exhausted that I slept for most of the week and gladly, through all of the side effects!

Chemo 5

I couldn't stop eating. It must have been the steroids that I was given to help boost the anti-sickness drugs making me hungry and I was ravenous; to the point that I woke up at 4am one morning and made a huge bowl of pasta!

Chemo 6

By this round I was completely bushed and I just cried in relief that it was all over, I cried non-stop for about 6 days!

'Chemo Coma'

'Chemo coma' isn't a medical term; it's something I made up to describe how I was feeling after the treatment was administered. Basically, it's like having the worst hangover you've ever had and

times that by 100 so imagine a hangover coma where you can't move, feel nauseas and exhausted; that's the 'chemo coma'.

This coma lasted for a few days after every treatment so during this time I had a family member or a close friend on standby, usually watching TV in the same room as me just to be there in case I needed anything i.e. a drink, food etc. Therefore I really think its important to have someone with her for a few days after treatment, no matter how insistent she is on not needing any help!

Preparing for Chemotherapy

Teeth

As previously mentioned, chemotherapy kills cancer cells and can harm normal cells and this can also include the cells in the mouth. Side effects can cause problems with teeth and gums, the glands that make saliva, the mouth lining and can also result in making it hard to eat and swallow. Therefore, it's important to see a dentist before starting chemotherapy to ensure that there are no other issues with the mouth and teeth and that they're healthy before treatment starts.

It's also important for her to keep the mouth moist to prevent drying out and getting sore.

How You Can Help

- Suggest she arranges to see the dentist about a week or so before she starts chemotherapy.

■ Ensure she has ice-cubes, ice-lollies and sugar free chewing gum, sweets or mints to help keep her mouth moist.

■ Have a packet of straws to hand; if she's finding it hard to drink due to the unpleasant taste in her mouth, straws can help bypass the taste buds!

■ If her mouth is sore, suggest foods that are easy to chew and swallow i.e. mashed potato, and avoid sharp crunchy hard-to-swallow foods also food high in acid like fruit juices can cause irritation especially if she has mouth ulcers.

■ Although the side effects can be unpleasant, make sure that she keeps her mouth, tongue and gums clean by:

- Using an extra-soft toothbrush to avoid discomfort.

- Brushing her teeth after every meal and at bedtime.

- Rinsing with mouthwash.

- Flossing gently every day (Avoid if the gums are bleeding and are sore).

My Experience

By fluke I went to the dentist with an infection just before I started chemo and I was told about the side effects on my gums. My dentist recommended that I have my teeth cleaned by the hygienist every morning before chemotherapy (Every 3rd week) and to also have antibacterial fluid

*injected in my gums to stop them getting infected,
with my immune system forecast to being low.*

*After finishing my treatment I had a number of
issues with my teeth and gums; my fillings came
loose and I had to have them all taken out and re-
fitted (All 8!!). My gums receded leaving my teeth
extremely sensitive and after trying a number of
different treatments; Corsodyl gel worked the most
efficiently and kept the sensitivity at bay!*

Mouth Ulcers

At the best of times, mouth ulcers can be quite a pain but
unfortunately the ulcers that appear during chemotherapy
treatment can be pretty awful, and big! The chemo can affect the
mouth lining causing it to get sore and resulting in these ulcers.

It's best to seek medical advice if ulcers appear, as there is
medication and a number of remedies available. I was advised
to gargle with salt water however as the side effects of the
treatment affected my taste, the salt water was insufferable but
I did find that swilling warm water in my mouth helped to soothe
the pain. Also drinking fluids through a straw can help her keep
hydrated and not aggravate those sores.

Infection

Infection is what happens when germs (i.e. bacteria, viruses
etc.) enter the body and multiply. With chemotherapy affecting
the immune system, she'll be more susceptible to catching

an infection so it is important to do everything to prevent infections or to spot an infection early and treat it quickly before it spreads.

Chemotherapy can make skin dry and if the skin is dry, it could cause the skin tissue to break, which is a great way for germs to enter the body and cause infection. Therefore it's important to keep the skin hydrated by drinking fluids and moisturising often with non-perfumed cream.

Mucous membranes line the internal body parts that come into contact with the air i.e. nostrils, mouth, eyelids etc. to ensure that they are kept moist as well as protecting against germs i.e. in the air, food, drinks etc. Chemotherapy can also damage the mucous membranes in the body therefore allowing germs to enter the body.

It's important to have a thermometer to hand; at the first sign of an infection take her temperature and if it's 37.5 or over, seek urgent medical attention.

How You Can Help

■ I actually read this morning (1st August 2012) on Twitter via @UberFacts that *'48% of fountain drinks and sodas are contaminated with E. coli'* so I'd suggest after reading that to keep her away from ordering any fizzy drinks off tap.

■ Keep a bottle of antibacterial fluid to hand.

■ Offer to help keep her house clean and sanitised.

- ■ To ensure she eats healthily and suggest upping her Vitamin C intake to help boost her immune system.

- ■ Make sure she has a thermometer and take her temperature daily.

- ■ Look out for signs of her feeling unusually warm, cold or flushed.

- ■ If she does get a temperature during chemotherapy, it's a medical emergency!

Nausea

This is probably the hardest section for me to write as recapping this part of the journey still today, makes me feel nauseous!

Chemotherapy can cause nausea and vomiting and unfortunately until she has her first chemotherapy, her Oncologist won't know which anti-sickness drugs are the best for her, as everyone is different. I've met women whose Oncologist chose correctly the first time and they didn't suffer any nausea at all. However, during my first chemotherapy the anti-sickness drugs had no affect at all and I had to be taken to hospital to be given an anti-sickness injection. Therefore I still associate chemotherapy with sickness (Hence me feeling rather peaky right now!).

For you to understand what I'm trying to say, let me tell you a quick story about when I was a teenager and drank too much of an aniseed-flavoured alcoholic drink that resulted in me being violently sick, and if I ever think about that alcoholic drink, I start to feel nauseous even though it was 20 years ago.

The same thing happened with chemotherapy but on a much larger scale as everything associated with it still makes me feel sick! This includes foods, smells and any red liquid i.e. cranberry juice, as it represents the colour of the chemotherapy fluid.

It's better to be prepared for this and for it to not happen than the other way around as it's not just the nausea, it's the emotion attached to the cancer journey as well. For example, is there a smell that takes you back to a memory or perfume that reminds you of a passed relative that can trigger the emotion of loss and sadness?

My Experience

I was advised to stop wearing my usual perfume when I was diagnosed so I excitedly spent an afternoon in a department store smelling perfumes and settling on a scent that reminded me of lemons. I wore this perfume pretty much every day from diagnosis until the end of my radiotherapy treatment, so in total about 8 months. A year or so later, I was walking down the stairs in my home when a whiff of that perfume hit my nose and my eyes filled with tears and I felt nauseas; my cousin saw the bottle on my bathroom shelf and decided to spray and smell it, sending a flood of emotions and sickness right through me!

On another occasion, a lovely acquaintance sent me a box of cupcakes that arrived the morning of

my second chemotherapy, which I fully indulged in.
Two weeks later another friend came to visit and he
too bought me a box of cupcakes however when
I opened the box, I started to feel really sick. That
feeling lasted over 2 years anytime I saw, or spoke
of a cupcake!

How You Can Help

- Make sure there are no strong smells around i.e.
  air freshener gels, plugins and sprays.

- Don't make her any of her favourite dishes to eat just
  after she's had her chemotherapy treatment – save
  them for when she's feeling better!

- Treat her to a new bottle of perfume.

- Buy unperfumed moisturiser and body wash.

Chemotherapy and Hair

Cold Caps

She might be brave and wear the cold-cap during chemotherapy.
These are hats, a little like horse riding helmets, which are filled
with fluid and frozen. When worn during the administration of
chemotherapy they chill the hair follicles, which limits the amount
of chemotherapy absorbed thus the hair doesn't fall out.

It can be a little unpleasant; remember the feeling when
you were a child and drank a frozen slushed drink which gave

you brain freeze? *Well to me it felt just like that, plus it's quite heavy on the head, so I took it off after 10 minutes and didn't wear it again!*

Hair loss

Hair loss for women is physically and emotionally uncomfortable and no matter how much you look in the mirror holding your hair away from your face, you can't ever imagine how it really feels to have no hair. And not just on your head but also losing your eyelashes and eyebrows, so it's important for you to help her keep her confidence up.

If you've ever had that experience of wearing a ponytail too tight and then once you've taken the elastic off you experience an unpleasant 'pulling' sensation, this is how it feels when your hair is falling out during chemotherapy, however this feeling lasts until all of the hair has gone. (For those of you who haven't ever worn a ponytail too tight, grab a small bunch of your hair now and pull it; the feeling is pretty much the same!).

If she were preparing to lose her hair, it would be a good idea to suggest she cuts her hair short before having chemotherapy for 2 reasons;

1. To get used to how it looks having hardly any hair so its not too much of a shock, as opposed to having longer hair.

2. The amount of hair that falls out is immense – so cutting it short would be easier to manage than scooping up clumps of long hair!

My Experience

I cut my hair into a short bob when I was diagnosed and then cut it shorter a few weeks later and then just before I started chemotherapy I cut it again, purely to make the whole process of losing my locks much easier to bear.

It's common for the hair loss to occur just before the 2nd round of chemotherapy is due, so about 2 weeks after the 1st round of chemotherapy, and it can last for about a week. *After a few days of hair loss I decided to shave it off as it became patchy and sore.*

How You Can Help

■ Buy her a satin pillowcase as she'll find it more comfortable to sleep on and it'll be less likely to cause friction on her scalp. *I wrapped my pillow in a satin nightdress instead of buying a pillow cover.*

■ Make sure she uses a gentle pH balanced shampoo i.e. those recommended for babies and children.

■ Advise against using a hair dryer or other heated appliances.

■ Suggest buying a wig before the 1st chemotherapy session so at the first sign of hair loss she can start to wear the wig (Wig shopping can be lots of fun so get her to try some colourful new styles).

■ Make sure she has a hat and/or a silk scarf.

■ To avoid the head getting dry, try rosemary oil together with a carrier oil (Preferably grape seed oil but you can use also a baby oil) and rub it on her head (Olive oil also works as a carrier oil but when I did it together with the rosemary oil, I ended up smelling like roast lamb!).

■ Shave her hair at home and not at a salon as not many female-only salons have clippers, so it could be embarrassing for her to go to a Barber Shop.

■ If you're Male and brave enough, shave your hair off too!

My Experience

I was given a bar of oiled soap from Lush Hand Made Cosmetics who recommended that I use it to help with the soreness of hair loss. I'd suggest going to your nearest store or another hand made cosmetic company and ask them for something to soothe the head during hair loss as it really helped me.

A breast cancer patient recently told me that her friends planned a girlie night out and they all wore pink wigs so she didn't feel self-conscious wearing a wig, I thought this was a great idea!

Eyebrows and Eyelashes

My eyelashes came out quite quickly however my eyebrows started to thin about 6-7 weeks into the treatment.

How You Can Help

■ Make sure she has false lashes and lots of glue.

■ Some cosmetic companies have great products to make the brows look thicker (Benefit Brow Shaping kit is great!).

■ Buy her a voucher for a Brow Bar – most department stores have them where professionals can paint on false eyebrows.

My Experience

I did have tears one morning when I woke up, looked in the mirror and my face was so dry from the chemo, my lips were cracked, I had a shaven head with patches of baldness and my face was swollen from the steroids...I didn't recognise myself anymore. It was frightening.

But remembering what my sister had told me before I started chemo, to 'Slap on some make-up, false lashes and my favourite clothes if ever I felt low'... and that's what I did, and I felt so much better!

Chemotherapy and Weight Gain

As treatment can affect people in different ways, she may or may not gain weight; some lose weight and some can get a swollen face/puffy cheeks during treatment. I'd say this is due to the amount of steroids she is given during chemotherapy so it's important to keep her self-esteem high as this can have a huge knock-on effect to her confidence, on top of losing her hair and everything else that goes with having cancer.

My Experience

I gained weight, just under 4 stone (That I'm still trying to shift!) however my swollen face went back to normal after a few months post-treatment. This was quite hard for me as the weight piled on really quickly so my clothes didn't fit and I felt very self-conscious with people I'd not seen in a while.

I'm not really sure what to say about how you can help, except to keep reminding her that these are just the side effects of the treatment, and if you're her partner/husband remember to compliment her and try your hardest to keep her self-esteem up as much as possible.

Chemotherapy and Exercise

I can't stress how important it is to make sure she's exercising during treatment. By this I don't mean sweating it out at a gym, but light exercises like walking. I read 'It's Not About The Bike: My Journey Back to Life' by Lance Armstrong (Truly inspiring book – I highly recommend it!) where he states that the morning before chemotherapy, he'd cycle for miles. Apparently exercising before and after chemo really helps in reducing the sickness (Something I learnt after my treatment so I never got the chance to try it out!). It's also important to ensure that there's a good flow of blood around her body, which will reduce the chances of blood clots and exercise is perfect for pumping blood around the body!

Furthermore, some believe that saunas can be beneficial as the cancerous cells are weakened in the heat; I'm not sure if this has been proven, but it can't hurt!

How You Can Help

- Plan a routine for the morning of her chemotherapy treatment i.e. that you take her for a walk through a park.

- Join a Yoga or Pilates class – joining together means that you can motivate her to go if she's not feeling up to it.

- Check with her Oncologist if she is able to use a local swimming pool. I've come across Oncologists who are happy for cancer patients to use pools however due to the risks of infection and the chlorine chemicals, some are hesitant to allow their patients to swim.

- Some local councils will give residents a leisure pass if they're out of work or on benefits. If she isn't working or has been signed off from work, check with her local authority as she may be entitled to free leisure facilities.

My Experience

During chemotherapy my body swelled and I gained a lot of weight and I was so exhausted that some days I couldn't make it up the stairs to go to bed! My husband would try to get me out of the house to walk around the block however I'd feel dizzy and couldn't wait to get back home to lie down. If I knew then how exercise could help in the recovery of treatment, I'd have walked every day!

Also an effect of putting on weight and not exercising meant that any time I felt pain, I was taken to hospital with a risk of blood clots which happened a few times and became quite a scary experience!

Chemotherapy and Monthly Cycle

If she is still young, there's a fair chance that her periods might stop during chemotherapy treatment however they should regulate about 6 months post treatment. It is also common that chemotherapy can cause early menopause in some women, unfortunately there currently isn't a way to know if this will happen and how to prevent it from happening.

If she's worried about fertility, make sure she discusses this with her Oncologist before chemotherapy commences to see what options are available i.e. egg freezing.

My Experience

I was told that I couldn't have my eggs frozen as my tumor was so high in oestrogen, so the fertility treatment was too much of a risk to take before starting chemotherapy. Some women choose to take this risk, I didn't.

My monthly cycle was regular throughout my chemotherapy but after the last chemo (Number 6), they stopped and returned about 10 months later. I had tests to check if I was still ovulating and was told that the hormone from the brain to the ovaries was quite weak. My monthly cycle can be regular for 2 months, then nothing for a few month so basically it's all over the place. But, something is happening so I've not hit menopause yet!

Radiotherapy

Radiotherapy is also known as radiation treatment and uses high-energy rays to kill cancer cells, decreasing the risk of recurrence in the breast. The treatment is given approx. a few weeks after the chemotherapy treatment has finished, or a few weeks after surgery if no chemotherapy is required.

Radiotherapy is usually given to only those women who have had lumpectomy surgery however those who had a mastectomy and had a high graded tumour, a large sized tumour or if cancer has been detected in the lymph nodes of the armpit, could possibly be given radiotherapy too.

Tattoo/Markings

To ensure that the radiotherapy rays are aimed directly to the affected area (And to not damage the healthy tissue) a tattoo of a small dot is placed to show the markings across the full breast area. This is so that when she goes for the radiotherapy treatment, the radiographer can align the dots under a laser beam line to ensure that the radiotherapy is applied to the same location every time.

> *I had (And still have!) a tattooed dot to the left hand side of my left breast, the centre of my chest bone and the right hand side of my right breast.*

Procedure of Treatment

In order to be given the treatment, she'll have to remove the top part of her clothing and wear a surgical gown and then lie down on a table underneath the radiotherapy machine.

One, or possibly two radiographers will position her underneath a 'straight line' horizontal laser, lining up her tattoos/markings. This procedure of aligning the tattoos/markings is done every time to make sure that the radiotherapy is applied to the exact area. Sometimes this can cause a little discomfort as her arms will be placed above her head, and the radiographer/s will shuffle her around until the tattoos/markings are perfectly aligned with the laser.

She'll then be left lying underneath the machine alone as the radiotherapy is applied, taking approximately 3 minutes, then she can get dressed and go home. It's advised to rub aqueous cream into the area every day after treatment to prevent radiation-induced soreness, see 'Side Effects of Radiotherapy' for more information.

The treatment is generally given over 15 days (Monday –
Friday over 3 weeks) at a hospital, and at approx. the
same time of day.

Side Effects of Radiotherapy

Her body will use up a lot of energy over the course of the
radiotherapy treatment, so rest is key as she may feel more tired
than usual.

She may develop a skin irritation in the treated area, this could be
that the area becomes tender, itchy, the skin might darken or go
red. Some women's skin in the affected area can become flaky
and dry like the effects of sunburn.

In extreme conditions, the skin could also split resulting in pain
and soreness so its really important for her to use the cream
given to her from the radiographer, which needs to be applied
daily, even if there are no recognisable side effects (This cream is
usually aqueous cream).

Other side effects could include shooting pains or swelling
in the breast area, which could last some time after the
treatment has finished. Again she need not panic; if she does
feel discomfort and a lot of pain in her breast, it is advised that
she does speak to the radiographer if this happens during the
treatment cycle, or to her doctor if the side effects occur once
the treatment is over.

How You Can Help

- It would be a good idea to take her to the hospital for treatment, as she'll start to feel the tiredness after a few sessions.

- The days start to feel like it's a recurring day, especially as the treatment is given approximately the same time every day, so I'd advise arranging a few fun, but not tiring, things to do after or before the treatment i.e. foot massage, cinema, afternoon tea etc.

- Make sure she rests! A nurse once told me that 'normal' people can get in from a hard day's work feeling tired, but get a 2nd wind to i.e. go to the gym, make dinner, visit friends etc. with radiotherapy, you don't get that second wind, so if she's feeling tired, she needs to rest!

My Experience

If you were to ask me 'What was the worst part of my cancer journey?' I'd say Radiotherapy, not the treatment itself, but the side effects.

I'd been given aqueous cream on the first day of treatment and was advised to apply it daily to reduce the side effects (Described as sunburn). After the first week of treatment I was examined by a nurse to ensure that the breast area wasn't sore or tender and she said to me that as I had olive skin,

I'd probably not be affected too badly by the treatment. I took this, as 'There's no need to apply the cream anymore', so I stopped.

The week after the treatment finished, I started to get pain in the breast and underarm area and when I looked at it, the skin in the armpit was purple and over the day it was spreading across my breast. By the evening I was vomiting and in agony and after a trip to the hospital I was told that this was normal and was given more aqueous cream and pain killers, and told to rest until it healed.

By the 3rd day the skin had split and my nipple has hardened and became burnt, the skin was so sore and I could only comfort myself by wearing sanitary towels inside a non-wired bikini top which was smothered in aqueous cream. I remember crying in pain as my husband had to apply the cream and he also said that this part of the treatment for him was the worse out of the whole cancer experience.

Therefore please remind her to apply the cream every day, even if the skin looks normal.

And please remember that cancer treatment can affect different people in different ways, hopefully she'll sail through it and this information was just a precaution!

7

Hormone Therapy

All breast cancer patients will be tested to see if their tumour had oestrogen receptors. This meaning that their cancer fed off oestrogen (The female hormone) in order to grow.

Depending on where you're from in the world, they monitor these results differently. For me, they marked the oestrogen receptors out of 8 and I scored 8 out of 8, meaning that my tumour grew only from the oestrogen hormones in my body.

As oestrogen is the necessary female hormone, it can't be fully blocked however there are a number of medications that can block cancer cells from feeding off the oestrogen and reducing the risk of the cancer coming back.

Receptors Explained

■ Oestrogen receptive tumours are known as ER+.

- If there are no oestrogen receptors on her tumour, this is known as ER-.

- If she is ER-, more tests will be given to see if her tumour tests positive for receptors with the other female hormone, progesterone.

- If her test then shows that her tumour was hormone receptor negative, then she won't benefit from hormone therapy.

Her test results will dictate whether hormone therapy is required and if so which is best prescribed.

My Experience

As I scored 8/8 for an oestrogen receptive tumour, I was given a 5 year course of hormone therapy medication Tamoxifen, which is a tablet taken every day for 5 years. This medication affects people in different ways however, most women that I've met taking this drug have had the same symptoms as I have; hot flushes, weight gain and tiredness.

8

Support

Other Ways That You Can Help

Have something planned for the end of her treatment to look forward to so it'll lift her spirits. I had a weekend in Venice booked, a friend of mine had an: 'I've finished chemo' party planned with all of her friends and family.

Gardening, although it sounds boring to some (Including me at the time!) is a great way to relieve stress, to give her something to focus on aside from the cancer and is also a great way to exercise (Just ensure she doesn't lift anything too heavy).

Although it'd be difficult, suggest she takes a photograph of herself at her darkest time. A friend of mine suggested it to me and said that if ever in the future I felt low, to look at the photograph and remember how far I've come and that things couldn't get any worse. At the time, I hated the idea and I've never told her this but I actually did it; I took a photograph of myself lying in a hospital bed; bald, grey skin and looking terrible, and I've never shown anyone! But I'm glad I did it and every now and then I look at the photograph just to see what I went through and what I'm now at the end of as still, I can't believe it!

When I was first diagnosed, a friend of mine suggested I choose a song to become my 'fighting cancer' anthem. So after a fun-filled morning of selecting the most appropriate tune, I decided on 'Eye of the Tiger' by Survivor, the theme tune to the film Rocky. Whenever I needed any encouragement I'd play this song, or if it came on the radio It'd make me smile (It still does!) and when I came through all of the treatment we sang this song at the top of our lungs at a karaoke bar. If there's a song that is personal to you both, or a song that you think will life her spirits, pop it on CD and tell her to listen to it anytime she feels the need for a boost.

They say that laughter is the best medicine, so make sure you have plenty of fun times!

Some Useful Information

Some oils (Including massage oils) are not suitable to use when she's going through or after chemotherapy, please seek medical advise before buying oils or having any spa treatments.

It's advised to not have any deep tissue massages up to 6 months after surgery.

When her hair grows back (Mine grew back curly even though I used to have straight hair!!) make sure she doesn't use any hair dye or harmful chemicals and to speak to her doctor to advise on when she can.

Check with her local hospital and cancer charities as there may be a number of complimentary events and therapies that she can enjoy.

Gifts

I've been told from a few cancer patients that they hated receiving a 'Get Well Soon' greeting card. Cancer can be unpredictable and no-one can guarantee survival even if the prognosis is good, so this type of card could upset her instead of making her feel better as 'Get Well Soon' cards are usually for people who are on the road the recovery.

> *'I just rip them up and throw them away as I can't bear to see them' a cancer patient once told me.*

If you do want to send a card, how about a 'Thinking of You' or a 'blank' card with positive words of encouragement and honesty? Say that cancer is hard, tell them that you're there for them whenever they need you to be etc. and if you are stuck for words, something simple like 'I just wanted to let you know that I'm thinking of you' is enough.

Great Gifts Ideas

- Magazine subscription
- DVD box set
- Comedy DVD or CD (Laughter is the best medicine!)
- Beauty items i.e. nail polish, false lashes, skin brush

- Sugar free mints, gum, sweets

- Non-perfumed shower gel, bubble bath & body lotion

- A new perfume or body spray

- Hire a cleaner for the duration of her treatment

- Journal or notebook for her to offload her emotions

- Something personal to help them get through the journey i.e. a special CD mix of happy songs

Why not make a hamper of goodies!

> *My favourite gift I was given was a t-shirt that my cousin stitched a handmade red and white heart on to; I wore it every time I had chemotherapy and it made me smile every time I put it on.*

Healthy Eating and Supplements

It's in our nature to panic at the thought of an illness and start pumping vitamins and natural goodness into our bodies when we think it's too late, and she will no doubt do the same... just try not to not let her go too much overboard!

How You Can Help

■ Investing in a juicer would be a good way to take in extra vitamins from fruit and vegetables.

■ If she insists on buying vitamins and supplements make sure she checks with her doctor to ensure that they won't interfere with her treatment.

■ There are lots of books and references available which advise on what natural foods can help heal the body (See the Appendix for a list of useful books).

My Experience

Like most post-treatment survivors, you feel like you're left in limbo; chemotherapy and/or radiotherapy is over and you're feeling a little lost and a little scared. No matter how grueling cancer treatment is, during it you feel like you're in a safety net, post treatment you realise that you're on your own...

After my treatment finished I started reading books and attending seminars about the natural ways to prevent and heal cancer so that I feel that I'm doing 'something' to stop it from happening again. As I said, I'm no medical expert, or even in the medical profession so I don't claim to be a cancer guru, but I thought I'd share my findings on what I'm doing in my new life without cancer and how you can include these little things into her diet.

Antioxidants:

Try to include a little bit of the following foods every day as they're PACKED with antioxidants:

- Apples

- Avocado

- Blueberries

- Broccoli

- Cinnamon

- Dark Chocolate

- Kidney Beans

- Lentils

- Mustard

- Oranges

- Oregano

- Raspberries

- Red Cabbage

- Walnuts

… and in case you didn't know… antioxidants protect your cells!

Beetroot is one of the key foods in preventing cancer.
The purple pigment has been shown to increase and normalise cell respiration – what I was told is that it helps to clone healthy cells only, so even if you had a tumour, it couldn't multiply as the beetroot encourages only good cells to grow.

I've bought beetroot capsules, which are good if she's not a fan of eating beetroot!

Chia seeds claim to be one of the most powerful, functional and nutritious super foods in the world!

They're full of:

- Fibre

- Antioxidants – apparently the highest antioxidant activity of any whole food!

- Protein

- Vitamins

- Minerals

… and is the richest known plant source of omega-3! Plus they keep blood pressure and blood sugar under control.

Pumpkins are a super anti-cancer food. One half cup of cooked pumpkin has over five times your quota for beta-carotene (Vitamin A0) per day. According to research at Tufts University it may be used to protect against many cancers.

Salvestrols exist naturally in fruits, vegetables and herbs however you need to eat organic produce to reap their benefits. Apparently they're like having a Police force in your body by transforming into chemical weapons that can kill cancer cells without affecting healthy cells.

You can buy Salvestrols in tablet form, I take 1 a day.

There are also a number of powdered grasses that you can buy where you just add a spoonful of the powder to a glass of water and drink. However there are so many of them on the market that I wouldn't know which one to recommend, so I'd suggest going to a health food shop and asking them to advise you.

They're great as they have high chlorophyll content which helps build healthy blood, transfer oxygen throughout the body whilst being full of nutrients, which help heal and regenerate the body.

The green powder formula can taste quite unpleasant so its best to either shoot it back or as I did, pour into a cocktail glass to make it at least look better!

How You Can Help

■ Pay attention to both of your diets. You don't necessarily have to have a lifestyle revolution to eat healthy.

10

A New Woman

On a personal note, I feel that coming through
the cancer treatment has changed my life,
however if I was told that when I was diagnosed,
I think it was a crazy statement to make!

But now I'm out the other end and I can see how it has
changed me; the cliché of having a 'new outlook on life' is
totally how I live my life now.

Some women go back to work as though nothing has
happened, some quit their jobs and change career, some
women go through depression from the shock of what they'd
just been through, and some, like me; feel lost in limbo!

How You Can Help

Research local group therapy sessions for women and breast
cancer so she won't feel alone in her 'new woman' thoughts.

If she wants to change her career then help her do it.

I mentioned before about how a holiday at the end of the treatment would help, so if you can, take her away so she can catch her breath and plan her fresh start!

My Experience

Post treatment I whisked myself off to New York; the place that I'd dreamt of going to as a child and never had the time to visit. There were times during my treatment that I thought of my regrets and not visiting New York was one of them, so off I went.

On returning from my trip I started back at work however the drive to and from work made me feel uneasy; it was because I had slipped into my usual daily routine as though nothing had happened, and I didn't like it at all. Even though I had finished treatment and people around me were saying 'At least its all over now', it was for them, but for me it was just beginning. The fear really kicked in, what I had been through was pretty tough and I was scared of the cancer coming back and worst of all, secretly convinced that it would come back.

I felt lost, I wanted my life to change direction and control it with my own hands, I needed meaning for my life and I scoured the Internet for days on end researching religions and spiritual retreats and also looking at courses in the local university prospectus to see if anything jumped out of the page that I'd be interested in. I felt desperate.

This is normal. Well now I know that, but at the time I was scared of my emotions, but looking back I can see how frightening and traumatic the journey of breast cancer was and instead of stopping, breathing and being grateful that I had made it, I panicked.

Appendix

Checklist

A few things to buy that might help you feel more prepared:

- [ ] Antibacterial gel
- [ ] Antiseptic Cream
- [ ] Dental Floss
- [ ] False lashes
- [ ] Grape seed Oil/Baby Oil
- [ ] Hat
- [ ] Head Scarf
- [ ] Ice-cubes
- [ ] Ice-lollies
- [ ] Moisturiser
- [ ] Mouth Wash

- [ ] pH balanced shampoo
- [ ] Rosemary Oil
- [ ] Satin pillowcase
- [ ] Skin Brush
- [ ] Straws
- [ ] Sugar Free Gum/Mints/Sweets
- [ ] Thermometer
- [ ] Unperfumed bathing products
- [ ] Vitamin C

Useful Websites

UK:

www.macmillan.org.uk

www.breakthrough.org.uk

www.cancerresearchuk.org

www.breastcancercare.org.uk

www.lilycentre.org.uk

USA:

www.breastcancer.org

www.cancer.gov

www.nationalbreastcancer.org

Australia

www.bcna.org.au

canceraustralia.nbocc.org.au

Useful Reading

It's Not About The Bike: My Journey Back to Life
by Lance Armstrong

*Say No To Cancer: The drug-free guide to
preventing and helping fight cancer*
by Patrick Holford and Liz Efiong

*What to Eat if You Have Cancer: Healing Foods
that Boost Your Immune System*
by Maureen Keane and Daniella Chace

The Breast Cancer Prevention and Recovery Diet
by Suzannah Olivier

Events

UK

Breast Cancer Care is a charity committed to offering support and information to those diagnosed with breast cancer. They offer a number of workshops including 'Headstrong', which is a private appointment to get advice and tips on hair loss, along with talks and courses across the country. For more information visit their website www.breastcancercare.org.uk

Penny Brohn Centre is a charity that offers a holistic approach for cancer patients including retreats, courses and support. For more information visit their website www.pennybrohncancercare.org

The Haven is a charity with centres across the county offering complimentary support and therapies including acupuncture and yoga plus information on nutrition and exercise. For more information visit their website www.thehaven.org.uk

UK & USA

Casting for Recovery is a charity that offers a fully funded retreat for breast cancer patients post-treatment where you learn and participate in fly-fishing, which can help build strength in the arm after surgery. For more information Google 'casting for recovery' to get the correct website for your country.

USA

Betty J Borry Breast Cancer Retreats offer a number
of fun adventure weekends and retreats for women living
with breast cancer. For more information visit their website
www.bjbbreastcancerretreats.org

Survivors Retreat offer a number of residential retreats in
Healing and Wellness and Sports. For more information visit
their website www.survivorsretreat.com

Australia

The OTIS Foundation Breast Cancer Retreats provide
complimentary retreats for both men and women living
with breast cancer. For more information visit their website
www.otisfoundation.org.au

Worldwide

Look Good... Feel Better is a charity that helps women with
the visible side effects of treatment. They offer complimentary
skin care and make-up workshops, even giving the cancer
patients a goody bag filled with high-end products! For more
information visit their website www.lookgoodfeelbetter.org

A Message for You

I really hope this book has helped you understand a lot more about breast cancer, and if it means that I've made just one person's experience easier to understand, then I'm a very happy woman!

Remember, there are lots of charities and organisations aimed at helping you through her breast cancer journey so use them, and meet other people who are going through the same experience as you are.

You can get through this and I'd love for you to get in contact and tell me if this book has helped you, plus if you have any comments or ideas that would make this book better for the breast cancer patient supporters of the future, contact me via www.katherineformosabown.co.uk

And remember, too many of us get caught up in our day-to-day lives to really appreciate life. So from experiencing this breast cancer journey with her should make you appreciate your health, and everything that's good about your life!

Katherine Formosa Bown

Index

NOTES

You gain strength, courage and confidence by every experience in which you really stop to look fear in the face.

Eleanor Roosevelt